I0843524

HOW TO REACH YOUR HEALTHY WEIGHT HANDBOOK

Maribel Ortells

www.comidasana.eu

Edition, layout and design by Plataforma del Autor, a Soul Goes Social, S.L. Trademark.

www.plataformadelautor.com

ISBN: 9781730968358

HOW TO REACH YOUR HEALTHY WEIGHT HANDBOOK

INDEX

INTRODUCTION

We could say, without being mistaken, that 99% of the people who are currently living in developed countries have followed a diet at some point in their lives.

Many of which, even though they've tried out many different diets, still remain overweight.

If we pile on the fact that there are diseases related to overweight, such as hypertension, diabetes, arthritis and cholesterol issues, among others, our worry increases and it's important that we do something about it as soon as possible.

These people go through numerous weight-loss diets only to abandon them in only a few months, just because they get tired of them or because they get bored with their meals.

The fact of the matter is that these people don't lose that much weight even after committing to the diet for several months, and they even get ill as a result of poor nutrition.

Obesity can be caused by many different things; it can be due to hormonal imbalance, mild hypothyroidism that has been wrongly diagnosed, malfunction of the adrenal glands, emotional problems we try to remedy with food, fluid retention due to food allergies and, of course, excessive eating.

Obesity is becoming a severe health problem in most developed countries; over 50% of the adult population suffers overweight, and child obesity is a growing concern, especially because children will suffer the consequences when they grow older, if we don't help them today.

Each country's government must help treat this disease, and it is calculated that about 5% of the health budget is going into the treatment of eating disorders such as this.

HOW TO REACH YOUR HEALTHY WEIGHT HANDBOOK

In this book I want to teach all of you how to better understand your body. Every person is different, and nutrition has to be personalized if we want our needs to be covered. That's why it's important to learn what kind of foods are the best for us.

I've split the book in two parts: Theory and Practice.

The theoretical part of this book will focus on basic concepts about diets, what it means to lose weight appropriately, the function of our metabolism, the impact of our blood type and nutrition, among other things.

All this theory is meant to provide a general understanding, so we can move on to the practical part of the book, where I share specific diets for each blood type.

Let's get started!

Maribel Ortells

THEORY

1. EDUCATING OUR CHILDREN

The statistics are truly alarming: 12-year-old children are not only suffering from obesity, but also from cholesterol issues, chronic fatigue, and rheumatic arthritis.

This is why it is important that we educate our children from a very early age about healthy and unhealthy food.

Well-nourished kids perform better at school, they are better at sports, and they are less likely to develop mental issues or disorders, as opposed to children whose nutrition is based on junk food, sugar, and dairy products.

Hyperactive children can benefit from a good nutrition as well. Symptoms can be relieved by avoiding certain foods such as wheat, dairy products, sugar, and red meat.

I want to share a very basic meal plan for children to start eating healthy.

If your child is diagnosed with a specific disease, you can contact me at www.comidasana.eu or via e-mail at info@comidasana.eu, and I will provide a specific diet to meet their needs.

BREAKFAST

Forget about dairy products and substitute them with a glass of vegetable milk, whether it is oatmeal, rice, quinoa, soy or millet. Serve it with organic whole grain toast and jam or whole grain cereals.

MID-MORNING SNACK

At this time of the day, it would be convenient to eat a whole grain sandwich with some protein; it could be soy, ham, pate or tuna.

LUNCH

Controlling what our kids have for lunch is not easy, specially, if they stay at school during lunch time. If they can come home or if you can pack them lunch, make sure they get some veggies, porridge, spelt pasta or rice and protein, preferably chicken or turkey rather than beef or lamb.

MID-AFTERNOON SNACK

They can have soy yogurt or a glass of vegetable milk with whole grain cookies.

DINNER

Their dinner should be light, so opt for some soup, mashed potatoes, mushrooms, asparagus, chard with yucca or sweet potato, and, if possible, fish.

Give them another glass of vegetable milk before bed.

I know that children and diets do not necessarily mix, and it will not be easy to make these changes. But, as parents, it is our job to try our best to provide our children with the best, most healthy options. If we succeed, common illnesses such as colds, asthma, otitis and obesity will be less severe on our children, and they can even disappear.

Here are some extra tips you can follow:

- You can make some French fries and other favorite treats from time to time.

- Do your best to remove all sweets from their diet and replace them with gelatin.

- If your children enjoy chocolate, we recommend that they have it in its purest form and without milk.

- Hazelnut cream can be replaced with carob bean cream.

- Breakfast cereals can be made of quinoa, spelt, rice, and they can even be chocolate-flavored or contain brown sugar.

- If they ask for snack bags, you can find organic yucca or potato chips, which are delicious, and they will not have a negative effect on their health.

- If your children love pastries, try to make healthy versions of them at home using spelt or light sugar, or buy them at organic stores. These products can be a bit more expensive, but if you think of the money you'll save on doctors and medication, it is definitely a good investment. For example, asthmatic children benefit greatly from a wheat- and dairy-free diet.

- If your child usually gets gassy around mid-afternoon, it is important that you eliminate gluten (learn more about gluten-free nutrition in the second part of this book) and dairy from their diet. You can easily follow any of the menus I provide in this book and increase their vegetable milk intake.

Eventually, children will get used to these healthier alternatives and the day will come when they will not ask for any other products, except the ones that make them feel good, healthy, and strong.

2. YOUR IDEAL WEIGHT

Now that we've talked about our children, it's time to focus on ourselves.

First of all, I want to show you how to find your ideal weight.

All you need to do is this simple calculation, known as Body Mass Index or BMI. "Calculate BMI by dividing weight in pounds (lbs) by height in inches (in) squared and multiplying by a conversion factor of 703.

$$BMI = weight\ (lb)\ /\ [height\ (in)]^2 \times 703"$$

Example: Weight is 150 lb and is 5´5" (6.5") tall, the result would be 24.96 ([150 ÷ $(65)^2$] x 703).

Source: www.cdc.gov

HOW TO REACH YOUR HEALTHY WEIGHT HANDBOOK

In the following chart we can see what the results of the calculation represent:

CLASSIFICATION	RANGES
Thin	Index below 10
Normal	**Index 20-25**
Overweight	Index 26-29
Type I Obesity	Index 30-34
Type II Obesity	Index 35-39
Type III Obesity	Index 40 or more

Discussing our ideal weight is actually very difficult because every single one of us has a different constitution.

The following tables are meant to serve as orientation to determine a person's ideal, healthy weight.

WOMEN

Size in ft	Narrow Constitution	Medium Constitution	Broad Constitution
5.16	103.84 - 110.90	109.79 – 117.73	116.84 – 126.77
5.24	104.72 – 112.88	111.77 – 119.71	118.83 – 128.75
5.33	107.36 – 114.86	115.96 – 121.70	120.81 – 130.73
5.41	109.79 – 117.73	116.85 – 124.78	117.06 – 134.70
5.49	112.88 – 120.81	119.71 – 127.87	126.77 – 137.78
5.57	115.74 – 124.78	123.68 – 131.84	130.73 – 141.76
5.74	118.83 – 127.65	126.77 – 134.70	132.72 – 144.84
5.81	122.80 – 131.84	129.85 – 139.77	137.79 – 149.69
5.90	125.88 – 135.80	133.82 – 143.74	141.76 – 153.66
5.98	128.75 – 138.67	136.69 – 146.83	144.84 – 157.85
6.06	132.72 – 142.86	140.88 – 150.80	148.81 – 161.82
6.15	135.80 – 146.83	144.84 – 154.32	151.90 – 165.79
6.25	138.67 – 149.69	147.71 – 157.85	154.76 – 168.87

MEN

Size in ft	Narrow Constitution	Medium Constitution	Broad Constitution
5.16	115.08 – 124.78	123.90 – 132.72	130.73 – 141.76
5.24	118.83 – 127.65	126.77 – 135.80	132.72 – 143.74
5.33	121.70 – 131.84	129.85 – 139.99	136.69 – 148.15
5.41	125.88 – 135.80	133.82 – 143.74	140.88 – 152.78
5.49	128.75 – 138.67	136.69 – 146.83	144.84 – 156.75
5.57	132.72 – 142.86	140.88 – 150.79	148.81 – 161.82
5.74	139.77 – 150.80	137.79 – 148.81	156.75 – 169.76
5.81	143.74 – 154.76	152.78 – 163.80	160.72 – 174.83
5.90	147.71 – 158.73	156.75 – 172.18	166.89 – 179.68
5.98	151.68 – 163.80	160.72 – 172.62	168.65 – 184.75
6.06	156.75 – 166.45	165.79 – 177.69	169.31 – 189.82
6.15	162.70 – 174.83	170.86 – 183.64	178.79 – 195.77
6.23	172.18 – 179.68	175.71 – 188.72	183.64 – 201.72

But, the main question is: how many calories does a person need in order to maintain a good health?

Usually, the focus of any specialist is based on the relation between our daily intake of calories and our daily expenditure of calories through exercise, work, housework, etc.

The problem is that some people eat very little, but they are overweight anyway. The opposite can also be true; some people eat whatever they want, and they do not seem to gain fat or put any extra weight.

This shows us that calories are not the only thing that matters; we also have to consider our individual metabolism.

Metabolism is the process through which our body keeps us alive. Our metabolism's efficiency determines whether we gain or lose weight, and how easy or difficult it is for us to shed those extra pounds.

The function of our metabolism is closely related to our blood type, so bodies with different blood types (A, B, AB or O) don't function the same way and the metabolization of food is very different for each individual.

3. The psychology of weight loss

Before we continue discussing calories and weight, I'd like to talk about the relation between our mental and physical state.

It's impossible to separate these two aspects of ourselves if we want to give our body a healthy weight, and more importantly, a stable health condition.

A person who wants to try a weight-loss diet must definitely be mentally prepared for the changes and the commitment. So, to reach that mental and emotional balance, we must achieve physical balance as well.

In order to maintain a good physical form, we must integrate physical exercise into our daily routine, whether it's walking, running, going to the gym, doing yoga, pilates, a sport, or any other kind of physical activity.

It is also important that we learn to breath consciously so we can calm our mind and control our cravings.

When we make our mind peaceful, our response to internal and external stimulation becomes more balanced over time. As a result, we feel better, more relaxed and we strive to transmit these feelings to the people around us.

It is important to understand that we are in control of our attitude towards life and everything we face.

A positive attitude is essential when it comes to recovering your health. Every aspect of your being should be in harmony: your spirit, your mind, and your body. If we achieve this, the rest becomes much easier.

Balance is very important in our lives and people who achieve it are those whose lives are molded to their needs, which is why they're happier.

4. When should we change our diet?

There are times in our lives when it is important to know the answer to this question.

However, before we can know this, we have to ask ourselves other important questions, such as: What do I expect to achieve with this change? How and when should I change my diet? How do I know I am doing it right? What can I expect from this?

1. You must change your diet at the appropriate time. Your body and your mind have to be ready for it.

2. The diet you choose must improve your health and help you find peace and harmony.

3. Your new diet must be pleasant, delicious and satisfying so you can feel good about your new eating habits.

4. Your new diet must make you feel focused, clean, and happy.

5. Your new diet must allow you to gain or lose weight, according to your needs.

6. Your new diet should also give you back your health if you have lost it.

The new diet must not make you feel:

1. It's a problem to organize your meals.

2. Depressed, bloated, stressed, tired, or keep you in a bad mood.

3. Confused or worried about the food you're eating.

When we change our diet we are essentially changing our way of life. Eating healthier means that we will have more energy to exercise, be creative, go out for walks, enjoy a book, enjoy sex, play with our children, and more!

In order to start changing our attitude towards life, we must practice habits such as these:

1. Exercising daily for at least 30 minutes. It does not matter what you do, as long as you get up and move. After a few weeks you will find that physical activity helps you relax!

2. If you do not want to exercise alone, find a buddy to join you or join a gym. This will make it easier to go out and exercise every day.

3. Give thanks every morning for being alive, for having a family and for everything that makes you happy. In short, give thanks for living!

These three simple steps are a great start!

5. Are all diets the same? Do they work equally for everyone?

No, all diets are not the same for everyone, and they can not affect everyone in the same way.

To understand why this is so, let's analyze a few things.

The first thing that we need to look into, is that we are living in an age where we are constantly advised to eat "healthy", but everyone has a definition of "healthy", so let's give this some thought.

Food in and of itself cannot make us healthy. A glass of milk can be deadly to some people, no matter how healthy everyone think it is in general.

Food is meant to nourish us without producing any kind of stress on the body. It must give us energy and provide what our body needs to heal itself and to keep us on the right track.

It's essential that we learn to listen to our bodies; not only listen, but also learn how to interpret the signs. Migraines, diarrhea, colic, and eczema, among others, are all warning signs that something is not right.

The following questions can serve as guidelines whenever you need to understand your body:

- Do you often feel confused, or lost? Do you forget things, or leave tasks partially undone? Do you trip over things? If the answer is yes, then it is possible that you are eating too many expansive foods (sugar, dairy products, fruit, and potatoes), which means you must change to a more contractive diet (green vegetables, legumes, fish, algae).

- Are you feeling uptight, stiff or inflexible? Do you have headaches? If so, it means that you are probably eating too many contractive foods and you're in need of expansive ones.

- When you wake up in the morning, do you feel a bitter taste in your mouth? This could mean that your diet is too acid, so try eating more alkaline foods (algae, fruits, vegetables).

- Do you binge on sweets after having a complete vegetarian meal? This could mean that your diet is too alkaline and poor in protein, so you must include legumes, whole grain cereals, fish and poultry.

- Do you often feel depressed and tired? It can be due to any of the reasons listed above, or maybe you are eating too much sugar or honey, so avoid these foods and include more fish and white meat protein to your diet.

As you can see, there are as many diets as there are individuals, so you have to find the one that suits your needs the best.

6. What should we do to start losing weight?

Sometimes a few small changes are all we need to help us lose those first few pounds, which are often the toughest ones.

Besides exercising on a daily basis, we must start a diet that will allow us to be healthy. Being in good health is more important than looking good, but we can accomplish both things at the same time; that's the beauty of good diets.

Not all diets are equally effective, not in all cases and definitely not for everyone. In fact, not all diets are healthy, and it is important that we tell the difference.

There are a few considerations you should always keep in mind to make sure your diet can provide good health and help you reach your ideal weight as well:

- On 99% of the cases, we get fat because we eat more calories than our body needs, on a daily basis. In these cases, the solution is changing our habits, which are often sedentary, and start exercising every day.

- We must accept the fact that we are all different, which means that no diet fits all.

- The best diet is that which is based on the changes we make on the table because that is where the truth about our ideal weight lies.

- There are still people who believe that, if they want to lose weight, they have to skip their meals, so they usually do not have breakfast or dinner. However, this is wrong! Our body reserves food in order to function until the next meal, so skipping meals can be dangerous. It is actually much better to eat 5 times a day, but we do need to watch our portions.

- Water does not make us fat, but it is better to drink it before eating, so it does not affect our gastric fluids during digestion.

- Light or Diet foods do not make us lose weight, and it is wrong to think that, just because they have less calories, we can eat as much as we like.

- It is very important to eat whole wheat foods with a high fiber content because fiber help us get rid of excess fat in our bowels.

- We must eat a variety of foods, but take into consideration that, if you want to lose weight, you cannot exceed the amount of calories you intake. I advise you to use smaller plates, so you can control your portions.

- It is important to understand that in order to control our weight, we must eat the foods that we really need. Avoid carbohydrates at dinner and snack on protein such as soy yogurt, almond yogurt, coconut yogurt or lactose-free yogurt.

- I think counting calories is out of place. It is far more important to live an active life, and eat regularly during the day; as much as 5 meals: three main meals and two snacks in between.

- Remember to include protein in every meal!

7. Must we starve in order to lose weight?

Of course not! As we've learned so far, losing weight is not only about removing certain foods from our diet. What is important is to meet our metabolic needs to the best of our ability and to exercise our body regularly.

For our metabolism to work as it should and help us achieve a healthy weight, it is essential that our body gets all the nutrients and enzymes it needs in the right amount.

The best way to achieve this is thorough a healthy and balanced nutrition. This means we must eat carbohydrates, proteins and good fats. We also must provide the right amount of minerals such as:

- Calcium

- Magnesium

- Manganese

- Copper

- Zinc

  And vitamins, including:

- Vitamin C

- Vitamin A

- B complex

- Folic acid and biotin

- Coenzyme Q10, which is very important for our body's functioning.

All these nutrients will allow glucose to metabolize in the right way, so it can have a good combustion.

This combustion allows our bodies to produce energy; if something goes wrong, glucose will turn into fat and accumulate in our body.

If food combustion does not happen as it should, the result is an accumulation of fat in your body and a low energy level, which can lead to chronic fatigue and overall lack on enthusiasm for our daily tasks.

This shows that when it comes to losing weight, stimulating and activating our metabolism is far more important than just cutting back calories and eating less than before.

In fact, diets that starve us and make us feel hungry all the time are easily abandoned after a few days or a couple of weeks, tops, due to lack of motivation.

What is more, these kinds of diets only work for a short period of time and eventually people get stuck and stop losing weight altogether. This is because diets like these slow down our metabolism in order to save energy, which makes losing weight that much harder.

For this reason, hypo-caloric diets do not work and, when we try them out, they only slow down our metabolism, which makes it difficult for us to eliminate fat, and they also make us very tired.

This is why it i's vital that we learn to eat healthy food in a balanced manner so we can enjoy our meals and never feel miserable about our nutrition.

8. Are carbohydrates and protein the best way to lose weight?

It is clear by now that our diet must be varied and it must contain all the foods that our body needs to function. But if we take a look at the most popular diets at the moment, we will find that most of them focus primarily, if not entirely, on protein. These diets eliminate carbs altogether, but this can cause a nutrient imbalance that will affect our health.

Lately we come across lots of advertisements for diets that focus only on consuming carbohydrates, in order to lose weight. The belief behind these diets is that carbs are healthier than protein, but none of these extreme diets are the solution.

It is true we need carbohydrates and protein, and they both must be included in a healthy diet, but it is very important to understand that not all carbohydrates or protein are healthy.

A diet that is rich in carbohydrates could be responsible for many of our present health problems, such as obesity, cholesterol, triglycerides, diabetes, menstrual problems, arthritis, and migraines, just to mention a few.

Carbohydrates can be found in: fruits, vegetables, cereals, grains, bread, pasta, flour, and legumes.

Having carbohydrates in our meals is important and nobody can say the contrary, but we must know what their glycemic index is, so we can choose those that are healthier.

The glycemic index depends on whether the food in question is composed of glucose, fructose or galactose.

Foods with the highest glycemic index are digested faster, so they make us fatter, such as:

*   Sugar, honey and glucose

- Dry fruits

- Bananas, grapes, figs, and melon

- Potatoes, beets, peas, corn, turnips, sweet potatoes, and cooked carrots

- White and whole grain bread

- Refined and sugary cereals

- Pop corn

Eating these foods will affect our reserve of body fat. In conclusion, carbohydrates are necessary, but they make us fatter than we think.

The best choice is to always get our carbohydrates from vegetables and fruits (these last ones must be eaten in moderation, due to their high sugar content) with low glycemic index.

According to my experience, the best way to lose weight in a healthy, long-lasting, and efficient manner is:

In case of obesity, where we must reduce a lot of weight, we must completely eliminate carbohydrates that come from:

- Grains

- Flours

- Legumes

- Bread

- Pasta

- Pastries

If we do not need to lose a great amount of weight, we can reduce the consumption of these foods to once or twice a week.

However, there are foods we must completely eliminate in both cases, such as:

- White bread

- White rice

- Pasta (not whole grain)

- Sugar

- Pastries

- Dairy products and their derivatives

Following these guidelines will allow us to maintain a healthy weight.

Remember to include protein in every meal!

9. Vegetarians and weight loss

For vegetarians, losing weight can be a lot more difficult because they have a limited food variety to play with.

Their diet is mainly based on a mixture of whole grain cereals and legumes, which is very limited indeed, but I can assure you that this one is one of the healthiest diets.

In such cases, it is recommended to reduce the amount of food we eat, increase our physical exercise, and lean more on tofu and vegetables for our meals. This means that vegetarians who have a lot of grains and flour on their daily menu will have to eat more tofu, protein and veggies if they wish to lose weight.

Soy, which is one of the main ingredients of a vegetarian diet, has a depressing effect on the thyroid gland. This means that it helps slow our metabolism down.

Vegetarians are also recommended to increase both fish and algae intake. These foods are rich in iodine, which serves to activate our thyroid gland.

I recommend vegetarians to follow a macrobiotic diet to lose weight, but I will talk more about that, later.

10. Fluid retention and weight loss

As you know, our body is composed of 70% water. Thanks to this water, and other substances, nutrients are transported through our body to where they are needed.

We have mentioned in the past that some people go through very severe weight-loss diets and they barely lose weight; well, the reason for this is that these people might have an excess of accumulated water, not fat. This is what's known as "fluid retention".

What could be producing this fluid retention?

- A diet low in proteins

- Nutrient deficiency

- Dehydration

- Food intolerance

Foods that may be causing fluid retention are:

- Coffee

- Tea

- Sugar

- Hydrogenated fats

- Salt

- Dairy products

- Wheat

- Alcohol

Foods that can help us with fluid retention are:

- Alfalfa

- Carrots

- Cucumber

- Corn

- Grapes

- Legumes

- Millet

- Turnip

- Algae

- Peas

- Pineapple

- Spinach

- Watercress

- Watermelon

- Pumpkin seeds

To get rid of fluid retention it is important to cleanse our body of toxins because toxin excess helps our body retain fluids.

My advice is to remove salt from your diet. If you find that you do not know how to cook without table salt, use marine salt or Himalayan salt instead.

11. Blood types and weight loss

After decades of investigation, Doctor Peter D' Adamo discovered the role that our blood type plays in the functioning of our body. His hypothesis is that each group, O, A, B, and AB has a different chemical reaction to food.

According to Doctor D' Adamo, there are molecules found in both food and bacteria called lectins, and these molecules have agglutinating properties.

When lectins travel through our bowel walls and into our blood, they react with certain blood components wearing our immune system down and causing harm to our organic system (liver, kidneys, stomach, etc.) while also attacking our white and red cells.

That's why the real solution to many autoimmune diseases is following a diet that allows us to cleanse our body, strengthen our bowels and increase our defenses.

Following Doctor D' Adamo's food lists, we will be able to improve our health in a simple and natural way. Each list is organized by blood type, so you have to make sure not to eat any of foods that are listed as not advisable.

This way, our immune system will not be worn out from fighting lectins, and it will be strong and ready to fight viruses and bacteria.

It is very important that we follow a diet that is perfectly tailored to our blood group because this will definitely help us lose weight a lot quicker and in a much healthier way.

<u>PRACTICE</u>

What you will find here

Now that we have reached the practical part of this book, here it is what you will find in this section:

- Because we have to take into consideration our blood type, I have decided to create a diet that will work for all different blood groups so that the whole family can adopt this diet.

- It is important not to obsess over the foods that each blood type must eat. Remember that these diets and lists should serve as guidance, but they are not set in stone.

- Your blood type is essential to understanding what your body needs, so you will find an explanation for your emotional and physical needs.

- We will learn about different cereals, especially gluten-free cereals.

- I will present the macrobiotic diet.

- I will also share some gluten-free dessert recipes.

Note: If you are intolerant to soy, whenever you find any soy food in one of these diets, you will have to replace them with a soy-free alternative. For example, you can replace soy yogurt with regular yogurt, preferably lactose-free, coconut yogurt or almond yogurt.

1. Blood Type "O"

People with this blood type are descendants of the first inhabitants of the earth, who were hunter-gatherers, and whose diet was based on fish and fruits. They can eat different types of meat, as long as their diet is balanced.

Cereals are not their allies and only rice favors them, but they must eat whole grain cereals like millet, amaranth, and quinoa. Wheat and dairy products are quite harmful on their diet.

They need regular physical activity, and in some cases, it must be very intense, so they can maintain a physical and mental balance.

These people can manage stress because they know how to face it and their attitude towards it creates the need to release hormones through intense and vigorous physical exercise.

Foods that favor weight gain for blood type O are:

- Cereals with gluten

- Corn

- Green beans, dry beans and lentils

- Cabbage, cauliflower and Brussels sprouts

- All dairy products

Foods that favor weight loss for blood type O are:

- Algae

- Fish and shellfish

- Meat, better white

- Fish, mostly for dinner

- Vegetables like broccoli and spinach

2. Blood Type "A"

People with blood type A descend from the first farmers, and because of this, their diet is based on foods such as oatmeal, spelt, millet, rye, fish, chicken, turkey, and fruit.

They tend to be quiet and calm people, so they need less physical activity, but they can run great lengths.

Their bodies react to stress by releasing adrenaline, which causes anxiety, irritability and hyperactivity. This causes their organism to weaken, which is why they feel the need to practice yoga, tai chi, martial arts and swimming, as a way to release stress.

These people shouldn't engage in competitive exercises or sports if they're feeling stressed because they will only drain their immune system, which can lead to sickness.

Foods that favor weight gain for blood type A:

- Meat

- All dairy products

- Common Lima beans

- Gluten

- Tomatoes

Foods that favor weight loss for blood type A:

- Olive oil

- Soy

- Vegetables

- Pineapple

- Gluten free cereals

3. Blood Type B

People with blood type B are a more evolved species because they can digest cereals as well as meat much more efficiently, but their diet must be based on turkey instead of chicken and fish, and cereals, preferably rice, quinoa and amaranth. They should also avoid corn, wheat and tomatoes.

Blood type B responds well to moderate physical activities, preferably group activities, such as walking, cycling, tennis, and relaxation exercises.

Foods that favor weight gain for blood type B:

- Corn

- Lentils

- Peanuts

- Sesame seeds

- Buckwheat

- Cereals with gluten

Foods that favor weight loss for blood type B:

- Green leaf vegetables

- White meat

- Eggs and fish

4. Blood Type AB

Blood type AB are a minority and they are the result of a combination between blood types A and B, so they have a mixture of positive and negative effects from both groups.

They feel good eating turkey, all types of fish, and whole grain cereals like rice, millet, spelt, and oatmeal. They should not eat wheat, corn, tomato and chicken.

If their intestines are inflamed, it is best to eliminate cereals containing gluten. They have a quiet character, so they require mild physical activity.

They react to stress much like blood type A, and when it comes to physical exercise, they must combine blood type B's mild physical activity with blood type A's relaxing physical and mental activity.

Foods that favor weight gain for blood type AB:

- Meats

- Beans

- Green beans/pinto beans

- Sesame seeds

- Corn

- Buckwheat

- Gluten

Foods that favor weight loss for blood type AB:

- Tofu

- Fish

- Vegetables

- Algae

- Pineapple

5. What is gluten and how does it affect your health?

Irritable bowel syndrome is a very common disorder and it causes a lot of discomfort. Sometimes this discomfort becomes anxiety, which we often mitigate by eating uncontrollably at all hours of the day, and this is one of the many ways we can gain extra weight.

If you feel anxious after your meals, <u>you must avoid cereals that contain gluten</u>.

The different diets I present in this book are all gluten-free, so continue reading to learn more about this.

Gluten is a protein that is found in wheat, oatmeal, barley, rye, and all derivatives, such as bread and pasta.

In time, gluten can damage the bowels of celiac patients and it also hinder vitamin and mineral absorption; this, in turn, can trigger a series of health problems, including fatigue and skin damage.

By adopting a gluten-free diet, you will alleviate symptoms related to these diseases. After a while, once we start seeing results, such as improvement in bowel health and nutrient absorption, we can decide if the patient can integrate gluten in their diet once more.

According to experts, celiac disease represents only a fraction of gluten intolerance, which in fact includes millions of people with less severe, yet problematic, reactions to the protein.

Even though celiac disease affects approximately 1% of the population, experts estimate that around 10% of people suffer a related condition which is poorly understood, known as non-celiac gluten intolerance, or gluten sensitivity.

Any kind of intolerance to gluten, including celiac disease, is often undiagnosed or wrongly diagnosed. This is due to its manifestation in different and complex ways, which can be confusing to physicians. Celiac and gluten sensitive patients usually suffer from stomachache, gas and diarrhea, which are the same symptoms of people who suffer from irritable bowel syndrome.

Celiac patients also develop headaches, tingling, fatigue, muscular pain, skin rashes, joint pain and other symptoms, as a result of the autoimmune warfare which gradually wears down the bowel walls, causing low absorption of iron, folic acid and other nutrients which affect everything, from energy production to brain activity.

"Gluten sensitivity is difficult to diagnose because celiac indicators are not easy to detect and there is no definitive medical analysis", says Daniel Leffler, doctor and assistant medical professor at Harvard University. People who belong to this group experience classical symptoms of the celiac disease, but they do not experience any detectable bowel harm and sometimes tests come up negative for certain key antibodies.

As you know, our immune system is in charge of fighting diseases, and the best way to keep it functioning is with an appropriate nutrition.

Having a healthy diet allows our immune system to remain up to task so we can transform our food into nutrients.

Cereals tend to unchain a series of rheumatic arthritis attacks which can cause swelling in our joints.

According to a British study, cereals, and more specifically cereals with gluten, were proven to be the main cause of disease in a group of patients suffering from rheumatic arthritis.

For this reason, I recommend you make the change to gluten-free cereals. Also, keep in mind that corn can also swell your joints even though it is gluten-free, so make sure to avoid this grain or eat it with caution.

6. Allergies and food intolerance

Food allergies are very common. There are some people who do not tolerate most of the vegetable milks on the market; I am one of these people. They make me feel really bad!

My solution has been making my own vegetable milk at home.

Needless to say, making your own milk is not easy, but it is definitely worth it.

You only have to invest in a machine to prepare vegetable milk, which is found both online and in organic food stores. Just be sure to compare quality and price so you can make the best choice for your budget.

These machines allow you to make vegetable milk from your favorite seeds and nuts, such as rice, millet, almond, spelt, or chufa, just to mention a few.

All you need to do is add water, and the machine will do the rest. It only takes 20 minutes to make around 2 liters of healthy milk.

Contrary to what many people think, drinking vegetable milk will not cause a calcium deficiency. Quite the contrary; if we eliminate dairy, we will become healthier.

In fact, we have to worry about losing calcium, but not about taking it. If our diet is varied and it includes a healthy variety of seeds, algae and veggies, and we exercise on a daily basis, our body will be healthy and strong.

Diseases such as Fibromyalgia, migraine, lupus, irritable bowel syndrome, chronic fatigue, arthritis and osteoporosis, all have pretty terrible symptoms, which can be relieved by the removal of dairy products from our diet.

Allergies and food intolerance are two different things. If you are allergic to certain foods, you will start feeling symptoms like throat swelling, headache and even vomit, within a few minutes or an hour at most.

Food intolerance manifests itself differently; here are the symptoms you should look out for:

- The symptoms will not manifest for a few days, or even a week.

- You may start feeling discomfort a few hours after the food intake, such as dizziness, cold sweats, migraines or stomachache. At first, it is not easy to recognize a food intolerance because the symptoms can be mistaken or taken as an isolated incident.

- If you start noticing these symptoms within a few days or weeks of following the therapy proposed in my book, it is important that you act quickly:

  - Make note of the time of day you felt discomfort, whether it is after breakfast, lunch or dinner.

  - Next, try to pin down the food that is causing said discomfort by making a list of all new foods included in your diet and do not eat them for two to three days. Discard them if they are causing the symptoms and remove these foods from your diet permanently.

You can also get tested at your local clinic to see what's causing the intolerance.

Remember that allergies and food intolerance can cause fluid retention, which means we will gain weight that we will not be able to shed with a simple diet.

Make sure you recognize your allergies and food intolerance and treat them accordingly.

7. Special occasions and meals

It is very important that we know what to do in special occasions when we're following a weight-loss treatment.

Many people decide to postpone the beginning of the treatment because they know they have a special event coming up.

However, this should not be an excuse to delay the beginning of your diet.

What this means is that you are not mentally prepared for the challenge of a new diet.

As you know by now, it is important that our minds are ready for the big changes and one of the many ways to start preparing is with physical exercise.

Suppose that you have already started your weight-loss treatment and one of your friends is getting married in a few days.

What should you do to enjoy the celebration without losing motivation or the progress you v've made?

To find motivation, just take a look in the mirror and notice all the improvements you've made so far.

To keep up with your progress, here are a few rules you should follow at any special event so you don't fall off the diet wagon and you enjoy yourself!

- Don't eat carbohydrates. Stay away from bread, pasta, etc.

- It's better not to drink during the meal, but if you do, opt for a glass of wine or water.

- Take bites of everything, but just remember: avoid carbs and turn to protein instead.

- You can have a bite of the cake for dessert and have it with a cup of coffee, no sugar or milk.

Once you're done eating, you'll want to get some exercise, so head to the dance floor!

If you follow these simple steps, you shouldn't worry about your diet during any celebration or special event.

If you have to go to important meals, such as work meals or meals with friends, here's what you should do:

All restaurants have dishes that contain veggies, rice, fish and meat, so make sure you order a salad and a protein such as fish or white meat with a side of vegetables (forget about fries!). You can order some fruit for dessert and have some tea or coffee, no sugar or milk.

8. Symptoms of changing your diet

When we change our diet, it is normal to experience certain symptoms, especially if we are adopting more natural, organic foods. Here are some of the most common ones:

- General tiredness

- Pains and aches

- Fever, chills, cough

- Abnormal sweating and frequent urination

- Acne, strong body odor

- Diarrhea or constipation

- Temporary decrease of sexual appetite

- Temporary cease of menstruation

- Irritable mood

- Restless sleep, slight hair loss, cold sensation

These symptoms may vary with each individual. It all depends on your health, and they can last from four days to a month.

9. Cereals with gluten and gluten-free cereals

Here is a list of cereals that will serve as an alternative for wheat.

As we discussed earlier in the book, wheat can produce intolerance, it can cause symptoms such as migraine, and it affects our intestines.

Not everyone has to eliminate gluten from their diet, so this list contains cereals with gluten that are healthy and beneficial.

OATMEAL: CONTAINS GLUTEN

Advisable for all blood types.

This food has been one of the main sources of nourishment for Nordic people.

It is one of the most complex cereals there are and it possesses high energetic and nutritional properties. The grains are set in such a way that natural elements such as light and sunshine, air, and water penetrate the plant deeply.

Oatmeal plants are only as high as half a meter and it is grown all over the world. It comes from Europe, where the plant can still be found in its wild form, and in America it is an essential food in everyone's diet.

It is a great way to reduce cholesterol.

MILLET: DOES NOT CONTAIN GLUTEN

Advisable for all blood types.

Millet has a high variety of nutritional properties but it is not as popular as wheat or rye because its properties and uses are ignored in many parts of the world.

Millet can be used for a great variety of dishes and it is safe for celiacs to consume because it is gluten-free.

Due to its low content of vitamin B3, millet has gained a somewhat bad reputation when it comes to diets. However, millet is not a problem in balanced and varied diets. In fact, it is a great complement for diets that do not focus on a single food.

Millet's vitamin B1, B2 and B9 content is greater than that of other cereals.

Millet is also ideal for athletes and people who practice extreme physical activity on a daily basis. It is also recommended for pregnant and lactating women because it is rich in iron.

RYE: CONTAINS GLUTEN

Advisable for all blood types.

Rye is a cereal that is rich in calcium, phosphorous and it has a high carbohydrate content as compared to wheat, and it contains less calories than other cereals.

Rye is a great cereal for making bread because it allows the bread to last longer and it is a lot more nutritional and tasty.

Rye is very helpful when it comes to weigh-loss diets because once it hits the stomach, it grows its size, making you feel full for longer.

AMARANTH: DOES NOT CONTAIN GLUTEN

Advisable for all blood types.

Amaranth is a wonderful cereal because everything can be used, both the grain and the plant itself.

In fact, amaranth leaves have a higher iron content than spinach. Additionally, they contain a lot of fiber, vitamin A, vitamin C, calcium and magnesium.

Some specialists say that we must boil amaranth if we want to use it as a vegetable because if they grow in dry soil, the leaves can contain high levels of nitrates and oxalates.

Amaranth also contains a high level of protein, as much as 15 to 18 percent. It also contains a good balance of amino-acids, which is not something you find in most cereals.

This cereal also contains between 5 to 8 percent of healthy fats and starch accounts for 50 to 60 percent of the plant's weight.

Amaranth seeds are rich in proteins, vitamins and minerals that help us grow healthy and strong. For this reason, it is a beneficial food for children.

Its high-content in calcium and magnesium makes it helpful for people who suffer from osteoporosis.

QUINOA: DOES NOT CONTAIN GLUTEN

Advisable for all blood types.

Quinoa is of great nutritional value thanks to its high protein content. This cereal provides all essential aminoacids we need to take every day, because our body is not capable of synthesizing them on its own.

Germ accounts for 30% of quinoa's weight and in most cereals, germ does not surpass 1%.

Quinoa is also gluten-free, which makes it very beneficial for celiac patients and people with irritable bowel syndrome and other intestinal issues and allergies.

Quinoa has anti-inflammatory properties, it contains carbohydrates, fat, protein, 95% of our daily iron intake and 12% or our daily calcium intake.

This cereal is also rich in amino-acids and it also provides vitamin C, E, B1, B2, B3 and folic acid.

When you compare quinoa with other cereals, you will see that quinoa is richer in calcium, magnesium, phosphorous, potassium, fiber, iron, and vitamin E.

10. Weight-loss Diet, Phase 1

Take a glass of kukicha tea with two tablespoons of chia seeds and let them steep for 15 minutes. Do this every day after you wake up.

Avoid adding too much table salt to your meals and you'll get used to eating this way a lot faster. Not to mention you'll avoid fluid retention.

Also, avoid eating more than one piece of fruit a day.

Breakfast	0.11 pounds of bread with (a different option for each day): • Spanish tortilla with asparagus and four olives. • Fresh cheese, preferably soy cheese, asparagus and four olives. • Tuna without oil, asparagus and four olives. Always take your breakfast with three-years tea. Keep the rotation going for a week.
Mid-Morning	One apple (if you suffer from gas, bake the apple or have apple sauce instead) with six almonds. If you still feel hungry, have some york ham, turkey and some tuna. Always take your mid-morning snack with some three-years tea.
Lunch	Always have some salad with Modena vinegar and Himalayan salt, carrot and onion (if there is something you do not like or makes you sick, you can remove it). **First course:**

	<ul><li>A plate of steamed veggies.</li><li>Mashed veggies. Avoid potatoes and have yucca instead.</li><li>Boiled yucca and green peas.</li><li>Legumes and veggies.</li><li>Whole wheat pasta (preferably rice, quinoa or millet) with veggies.</li></ul> You can choose among these dishes and rotate every day. **Second course:** Some white meat; chicken, turkey or pork.
Mid-afternoon	If you get hungry, have some turkey, york ham or tuna. Choose between: Soy yogurt or lactose-free milk. One avocado with Serrano ham. One piece of fruit. Always take your mid-afternoon snack with some three-years tea.
Dinner	<ul><li>Grilled veggies or mashed veggies, mushrooms, and asparagus.</li><li>Grilled fish fillet.</li><li>Chicken or tofu burger.</li><li>An infusion.</li></ul> Avoid oil and use little to no salt.

Follow this diet for four weeks.

11. Weight-loss Diet, Phase 2

Take a glass of kukicha tea with two tablespoons of chia seeds and let them steep for 15 minutes. Do this every day after you wake up.

Avoid adding too much table salt to your meals and you'll get used to eating this way a lot faster. Not to mention you'll avoid fluid retention.

Also, avoid eating more than one piece of fruit a day.

Breakfast	0.17 punds of gluten-free bread with (choose a different option every day): • Spanish tortilla with asparagus and four olives. • Fresh cheese, preferably soy cheese, asparagus and four olives. • Tuna without oil, asparagus and four olives. • Teff cereals with sesame seeds of 0.11 pounds of teff and vegetable milk. Always take your breakfast with three-years tea. Keep the rotation going for a week.
Mid-Morning	One apple (if you suffer from gas, bake the apple or have apple sauce instead) with six almonds. If you still feel hungry, have some york jam, turkey and some tuna. Always take your mid-morning snack with some three-years tea.
Lunch	Always have some salad seasoned with Modena vinegar and Himalayan salt and add carrots and onion (if there is something you do not like or makes you sick, you can remove it). First course:

	• A plate of steamed or grilled veggies. • Mashed veggies. Avoid potatoes. • Boiled green peas and yucca. • 0.13 pounds of quinoa, brown rice, millet, or amaranth with veggies. • Legumes and veggies. • Whole wheat pasta (preferably rice, quinoa or millet) with veggies. You can choose between these dishes and rotate every day. Second course: Some white meat; chicken, turkey or pork.
Mid-Afternoon Snack	Choose between: • Soy yogurt or lactose-free milk. • One avocado with Serrano ham. • One piece of fruit. Always take your mid-afternoon snack with some three-years tea.
Dinner	• Grilled veggies or mashed veggies, mushrooms, and asparagus. • Grilled fish fillet. • Chicken or tofu burger. • Grilled or baked white meat. • Veggie or tofu burger. • An infusion. Avoid oil and use little to no salt. Follow this diet for four weeks.

Follow this diet until you reach your ideal weight.

12. How your nutrition should be to maintain your health and your ideal weight

Before you have breakfast, take kukicha tea and let chia seeds steep in the tea for ten minutes until they soak it up.

Breakfast	Choose between these two breakfast options: 1. Kukicha tea with two toasts, 0.17 pounds of rice bread, vegetable pate, cold turkey and Serrano ham. 2. Soy milk, sugar-free almonds, 0.13 pounds of sugar-free rice cereal, amaranth, quinoa, and tapioca with a teaspoon of pure cocoa or coffee and stevia.
Mid-Morning	If you need more calories, you can have one fruit or two toasts of gluten-free bread with protein. An infusion with stevia and six raw almonds.
Mid-Afternoon Snacks	Soy yogurt or a glass of vegetable milk with two gluten-free cookies.

The following diet is meant to help you understand how your weekly menu should be like. Avoid eating carbohydrates at night.

	Lunch	**Dinner**
Monday	• Salad • Lentils or azukis • One chicken hamburger with gluten-free bread	• Veggie cream, mashed zucchini with onion, salt and olive oil • Sole • Relaxing infusion
Tuesday	• Salad, steamed broccoli and turkey • 25gr of rice bread • One infusion with stevia	• Asparagus with salmon • Relaxing infusion
Wednesday	• Salad • Brown rice with baked veggies and chicken (baked rice) • Infusion	• Steamed cabbage • Grilled trout • Relaxing infusion
Thursday	• Quinoa with veggies and/or legumes • Egg with gluten-free bread • Infusion	• Asparagus • Mushroom stir • Veggie burger
Friday	• Salsa • Whole wheat macaroni with tuna or diced turkey • Sauteed onions and broccoli	• Veggie and mushroom tortilla. • Infusion with stevia.
Saturday	• Salad • Chicken broth with veggies and rice noodles • Sea bass	• Gluten-free pizza with veggies, tuna and onions.
Sunday	• Varied salad • Rice with beef and veggies • Homemade	• Veggie stir • Veggie or fish burger • Relaxing infusion

13. Recipes

Now we have come to the fun part!

These recipes are all super easy to make and they are very nutritious as well. They are perfect to help you follow your diet!

<u>Cereal Recipe</u>

Ingredients:

- 0.04 pounds of millet seeds

- 0.04 pounds of quinoa seeds

- 0.04 pounds of amaranth seeds

- 1 tablespoon of raw sesame seeds

- 1 tablespoon of tapioca grits

- Soluble coffee

Preparation:

Put all the ingredients in a boiling pan and add equal parts of vegetable almond milk and water.

Add stevia or coconut sugar to taste.

Boil for 15 minutes and stir occasionally.

You can make this at night and heat it up in the morning.

Brown Rice Bread

This is a very special recipe. The majority of my patients love it because they will be using brown rice flower to make gluten-free bread at home.

The flavor will be softer, sweeter and it goes well with any kind of food. You can use this bread to make gluten-free snacks with sugar-free marmalade, vegetable pate, have toasts with fried eggs, and anything else you can think of.

To get started, we need to prepare the yeast. Follow this recipe:

Yeast Recipe

Grab a crystal bowl with a lid and make a hole on the lid so that the gas can escape. All you need for this is brown rice flour and water.

The preparation takes 4 days, here it is what you will have to do:

Day 1: Fill the bowl with equal parts of water (at room temperature) and flour. Do not overfill the bowl, stir everything together and let it rest for a day.

Day 2: Throw away half of the dough and add equal parts of flour and water so that you fill the bowl just like the day before. Stir everything well and let it rest for a day. Mark the size of the dough so you can see the difference the next day.

Day 3: The dough should be significantly swollen and full of bubbles. The level should have risen 0.78 inches above the mark you made on day 2. Throw away half of the dough and refill the bowl with equal parts of flour and water.

Day 4: If everything goes well, the yeast is ready to use! You can store it in the fridge and continue to add flour and water every day.

Rice Bread

Ingredients:

- 99 pouns of gluten-free brown rice flour
- Half a liter of tepid water
- A pinch of Himalayan salt
- 3 tablespoons of yeast

Preparation:

1. Add the flour, the salt, the yeast and the water in a bowl.
2. Stir everything until you have a thick dough.
3. Cover the dough with a cloth and let it rest for 4 to 5 hours until it doubles its size.
4. Work the dough with your hands.
5. Fill your molds.
6. Preheat the oven at 210 degrees celcius and bake your bread for an hour or until it browns. If you move the mold and the bread does not stick to it, then it is done.
7. Take it out of the oven once it is ready, unmold and let it rest.

You can use this dough to make gluten-free pizza as well!

Special desserts that do not make us fat

All diets allow for a cheat day or a special day. My special day is Friday night, so I pick a good movie and I get comfy on my couch with a cup of hot chocolate to enjoy some "me time". We all have our special moments and we can spend them alone or in the company of others.

I recommend that you create such a moment for yourself once a week. Choose a food that makes you happy and just enjoy your meal and your day!

Here are a few ideas for guilt-free desserts. They do not have many calories and they are delicious!

If you do not have a sweet tooth, just choose your favorite food and enjoy your cheat day anyway.

<u>Cheese and strawberry mousse</u>

Ingredients:

- 0.55 pounds of fresh cheese (or soy cheese)

- 2 eggs whites

- 3 tablespoons of fructose

- 0.22 pounds of raspberries

- 0.22 pounds of strawberries

Preparation:

1. Beat egg whites until stiff, add 1 tablespoon of fructose.

2. Mix fresh cheese with the other 2 tablespoons of fructose and add the egg whites carefully until we obtain a mousse.

3. Cut fruit in small pieces and add them.

4. Place in a bowl and put in the fridge for a few hours.

Cookie Pie

Ingredients:

- 1 pack of cookies Maria type (0.22 pounds) smashed

- 0.55 pounds of sugar free strawberry jam

- 2 and ½ tablespoons of unflavored powdered gelatin or 5 gelatin sheets

- 2 strawberry skimmed yogurts

- 2 tubs of diet creamy cheese (Philadelphia type), or soy spread

- 1 and ½ cups of strawberry pieces

- 25 drops of liquid sweetener (you can also use it powdered)

Preparation:

1. Mix smashed cookies with strawberry jam and cover the bottom of a detachable cake pan.

2. Dissolve powdered gelatin in half cup of hot water and leave it until warm. Mix yogurt with cheese and strawberry pieces. Add slowly the warm gelatin, the sweetener and mix well.

3. Finally, drop the mix in the mold where we have the smashed cookies, and put it in the fridge for about 30 minutes until it thickens. It must be served cool.

<u>Chocolate cake</u>

Ingredients:

- 0.55 pounds of pure chocolate without milk

- 5 eggs

- 1 teaspoon of orange peel

- 1 pinch of salt

- 2 tablespoons of brandy

Preparation:

1. Melt the chocolate.

2. Separate egg whites from the yolks. Beat egg whites until stiff adding a pinch of salt.

3. Mix the chocolate with the brandy and half of the orange peel and stir until mixed well.

4. Let cool for 2 or 3 minutes and mix it with the egg yolks.

5. Add the beaten egg whites and mix. Drop the mixture into a cake mold. It must be about 2 inches thick.

6. Add on the top the rest of the orange peel. Bake for 20 minutes in preheated oven at 100º C

<u>Chocolate mousse</u>

Ingredients for 4 people:

- 0.28 pounds of black chocolate

- Vegetable milk, of rice, oatmeal, soy…

- 3 egg yolks

- 4 egg whites

- 3 tablespoons of brown sugar

- 0.16 pounds of soy margarine

- A bit of salt

Preparation:

1. Cut up the chocolate and put in a pot with the milk until it melts. Then add the margarine, also in pieces.

2. Meanwhile, beat the egg whites until stiff and add a bit of salt.

3. When the chocolate, milk mixture cools down, add the beaten egg whites, stirring carefully. Add the egg yolks.

4. When the color of the mixture gets even and spongy, we let it rest, and put in four containers.

5. Let it cool down and put it in the fridge for 2 hours at least. In the winter, there are people who also eat it warm.

6. These recipes are courtesy of Sabores.com. Nutrition that gives you back your lost health!

Rice Flour Biscuit

Ingredients:

- 4 eggs

- 4 tablespoons of rice molasses

- 1 glass of vegetable milk

- 1 pack of baking powder

- 3 tablespoons of olive oil

- 1 pinch of Himalayan salt

- 1 lemon peel

Preparation:

1. Mix ingredients in a bowl, eggs, vegetable milk, molasses, baking powder and salt. Stir well. Add lemon peel, oil and finally flour. Mix well with a spoon.

2. Put in the oven at 175ºC during 30 minutes or until it gets golden.

This is a great choice for breakfast, mid-afternoon snack and dessert!

Tip: We can prepare a dessert with this biscuit adding some dark chocolate spread of 80% cocoa.

<u>Gipsy's Arm with whole grain flour</u>

Ingredients:

For the biscuit:

- 0.26 pounds of whole grain brown sugar

- 0.26 pounds mixture of brown rice and corn flours

- 3 eggs

- One lemon peel

For the filling:

- Chocolate spread or carob cream

- Strawberry jam

- Ground cinnamon

- Almond or hazelnut flour

Preparation:

1. Beat the egg whites until stiff, add the brown sugar and beat again. Add egg yolks, flour and lemon peel.

2. Extend the dough on oven paper in an oven tray and bake during 10 minutes.

3. Separate the dough from the paper before it cools down.

To fill the biscuit:

1. We can use carob cream, chocolate spread or the chocolate from the previous recipe.

2. Carob cream does not contain milk and the sugar used in it is brown sugar. We can decorate it with strawberry jam. I put on top some ground cinnamon or almond flour.

3. We must roll the dough very carefully, it will not look as perfect as the ones sold in pastry stores, but it will be just as tasty, and a lot healthier.

14. The nutrition that gives you back your lost health

What does the Macrobiotic diet consist of?

Long lasting life. This is the definition that George Oshawa gives to this way of nourishing our body.

The macrobiotic diet is based on the belief that we must take into consideration several aspects of life in order to determine a perfect eating style. Weather, work, geographic location and health condition are some of the main aspects to consider.

Long-lived life, but also a full and happy life. This is a Macrobiotic feeding.

I have been following this diet for some time now and, do you know what I have noticed ever since I started eating like this? A feeling of fulfillment! I feel how my body heals from the inside, specially my bowels. Ever since I was little, I have always suffered of irritable bowels, and this diet has finally given me comfort.

This feeling of internal healing is one of the effects of following the macrobiotic diet; limiting your meat intake or eliminating it entirely, and eating whole grain cereals and legumes, which sooth our nervous system thanks to the vitamin B they provide, is extremely beneficial.

When we eliminate expansive foods like sugar, excess fruit, juices and salads, we feel better and our body, specially our bowels, starts to repair itself.

Experiencing bowel swelling can cause symptoms such as restlessness, anxiety, tiredness, and we simply feel bad. In turn, this can cause our irritable bowel symptoms to aggravate, including intestinal gases, diarrhea or constipation, bad mood, headaches, migraines and weight gain.

Many people who follow a macrobiotic diet have a remission or disappearance of diseases like Fibromyalgia, chronic fatigue, irritable bowel, migraine, arthritis and osteoporosis, lupus, and even cancer. This is because healthy bowels allow us to prevent and treat this kind of diseases.

But not everybody can follow a strict macrobiotic diet; some people get ill, specially group O patients.

I know many of you will not believe this, but I have been a nutritionist for many years and I have treated people with different blood groups. My experience has allowed me to determine that group O individuals who insist in being vegetarians or following a macrobiotic diet, just cannot go through it. Some patients in this group absolutely have to include white meat to their macrobiotic diet at least two or three times a week.

Why does this happen?

Well, remember that people with blood group O descend from hunter-gatherers and they benefit a lot more from a nutrition based on meat. Additionally, they do not metabolize vegetable protein from cereals and legumes correctly, so they have to choose the right kind of cereals and legumes for their metabolism.

I have decided to take it a little bit further in my therapy and I have linked several concepts together to create a gluten-free macrobiotic diet that is easier to understand and to follow, and that won't hurt your budget either. What I do is include gluten-free cereals and flours into the diet, leaving standard cereals and flours out of the picture.

Which gluten-free, healthy cereals can we include in this diet?

- Millet

- Soy

- Amaranth

- Quinoa

- Rice

- Corn, but this one with caution

On top of cereals, we can add legumes, vegetable milk made from the aforementioned cereals, fish (twice or three times a week), algae, eggs (once a week), homemade rice bread, etc.

Believe it or not, many of you are unconsciously following a macrobiotic diet, because you want to improve your physical and emotional condition.

The macrobiotic diet allows us to find inner peace and calm, which we can apply to our everyday life, and it also allows our body to heal. Imagine what would happen if the whole world would adopt this diet? Life would improve greatly!

An appropriate nutrition would allow us to prevent and heal many diseases and eliminate health care and pharmacological expenses from our lives. This is what the macrobiotic diet has to offer.

All the diets I propose in my books are healthy and they help prevent, treat, and cure the diseases that threaten our lives all over the world.

Here are other facts about the macrobiotic diet so you can learn even more:

- The Macrobiotic diet does not produce anemia. Meat is not the only source of iron. In fact, other foods produce iron that is easier for our bodies to assimilate. For example, alga spirulina. If you include these algae in your diet, you'll never have any iron-related issues.

- The Macrobiotic diet does not decalcify us. On the contrary, when we replace the foods that eliminate calcium from our diet, we do not have to worry about it anymore. Foods that remove calcium from our body are, among others, dairy products and sugar. If we include whole grain cereals, vegetables and algae, we will not have to worry about calcium deficiency.

- The Macrobiotic diet does not undernourish or dehydrate our boy; the diet includes fluids such as tea and soups, and water intake is encouraged on a daily basis.

- The Macrobiotic diet should not limit our social activities and it should not be a hindrance in our social interactions. It is very easy to find dishes that work for the macrobiotic diet in any restaurant, so it should not be a problem. Most restaurants offer vegetarian and seafood options, so there is no reason to make a mountain out of a mill hole.

It is important that we do not go to extremes with any kind of diet! Extremes are bad in every aspect of our lives, so be careful not to overdo it. Your diet should not make your life harder, it should only improve it and make you happy by allowing you to accomplish your goals.

15. Macrobiotic Diet

Take 2 spirulina pills, 2 magnesium pills and a glass of warm water with a bit of Himalayan salt on an empty stomach every day before breakfast.

Breakfast

4 days a week:

- Millet cream, quinoa and amaranth, boil a tablespoon of each in two glasses of water for 20 to 25 minutes.

- Three-years tea.

3 days a week:

- One cup of malt, cereal, coffee or three-year tea.

- And alternate the following:

  - Rice waffle with 100 % fruit jam.

  - Toasted rice bread with olive oil.

  - Muesli without sugar, rice or corn cereal flakes with vegetable milk.

Mid-afternoon snack

- 1 glass of vegetable milk, soy, rice, quinoa, almond, millet.

- Rice bread toast or rice flour biscuit.

Lunch	**Monday and Thursday**	<ul><li>Pumpkin and onion soup, we can add miso</li><li>Millet with cauliflower and onion</li><li>Garbanzo beans with parsley and carrots</li></ul>
Dinner	**Monday and Thursday**	<ul><li>Onion soup with algae and miso</li><li>Rice spaghetti</li><li>Vegetable stew</li></ul>
Lunch	**Tuesday and Friday**	<ul><li>Julienne soup with vegetables and algae</li><li>Rice macaroni with vegetables and seitan</li></ul>
Dinner	**Tuesday and Friday**	<ul><li>Fish soup with arame algae</li><li>Mushroom, onion and brown rice stew</li></ul>
Lunch	**Wednesday**	<ul><li>Lentil soup with miso</li><li>Brown rice with cooked vegetables, turnip, carrots and onion</li></ul>
Dinner	**Wednesday**	<ul><li>Cauliflower and onion soup</li><li>Millet nuggets with onion, leeks and carrots</li></ul>
Lunch	**Saturday**	<ul><li>Carrot cream</li></ul>

		• Millet with vegetables • Steamed or grilled fish
Dinner	**Saturday**	• Miso soup with garbanzo beans • Spaghetti with vegetables • Vegetable stew
Lunch	**Sunday**	• Brown rice with vegetables • Azukis with algae and pumpkin • Miso soup with algae
Dinner	**Sunday**	• Carrot cream • Millet with vegetables • Steamed or grilled fish

It is important that you learn to prepare your meals in advance, so you save time!

Now that we have learned all this new information, I have to point out that each person is different, so there are factors to take into consideration when treating different diseases.

It is important that each one of you has a personalized diet while following the guidelines I provide in this book to achieve a healthy and full life.

This diet is meant for those who want to make a radical change in their lives. It is really a very healthy way of eating, it prevents diseases, it detoxifies the body and it helps you lose weight.

If you notice any symptoms, make the changes necessary to your diet and please consult a physician.

Other books by Maribel Ortells that might interest you

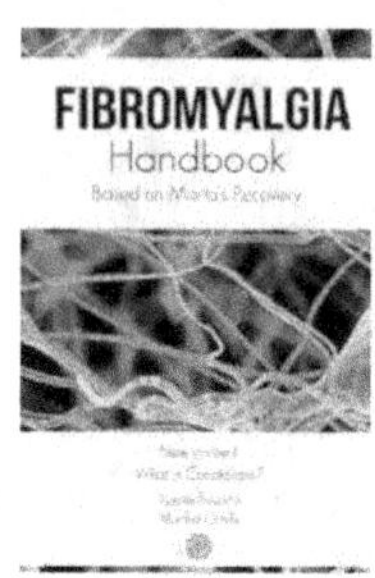

In this book, Maribel Ortells contributes her personal experience in the treatment and reduction of the symptoms caused by Fibromyalgia.

With this manual you can understand what is causing the symptoms, and how through a specific diet, you can begin to live without pain and feel better.

Based on her own daughter experience, Maribel explains you how her family started fighting to reduce Fibromyalgia symptoms until her daughter became able to have a life with no pain.

This book is available in Amazon.com

BIBLIOGRAPHY

- "Blood groups and nutrition"

  Authors: Peter D'Adamo and Catherine Whitney

  Editor: Javier Vergara

- "Balance through nutrition"

  Author: Olga Cuevas Fernández

  Editor: Sorles S.L.

- "Orthomolecular nutrition"

  Author: Cala H Cervera

  Editor: Robin Book

- "The healing power of food"

  Author: Annemarie Colbin

  Editor: Robin Book

- "Your erroneous zones"

  Author: Wayne W. Dyer

  Editor: Debolsillo clave

- "Biological Medicine"

  Author: Txumari Alfaro

  Editor: Ediciones B, for Zeta de bolsillo

- "Fibromyalgia handbook" Based on Marta's Recovery

  Authors: Maribel Ortells and Vicente Estupiñá

  Editor: Carena Editors

- "Recover your health with nutrition"

  Author: Maribel Ortells

  Editor: Carena Editors

  Others:

- Sabores.com (Flavors.com)
- Manual de Fibromialgia (Fibromyalgia Handbook)

www.comidasana.eu

www.ingramcontent.com/pod-product-compliance
Lightning Source LLC
Chambersburg PA
CBHW061710250726
48657CB00002B/586